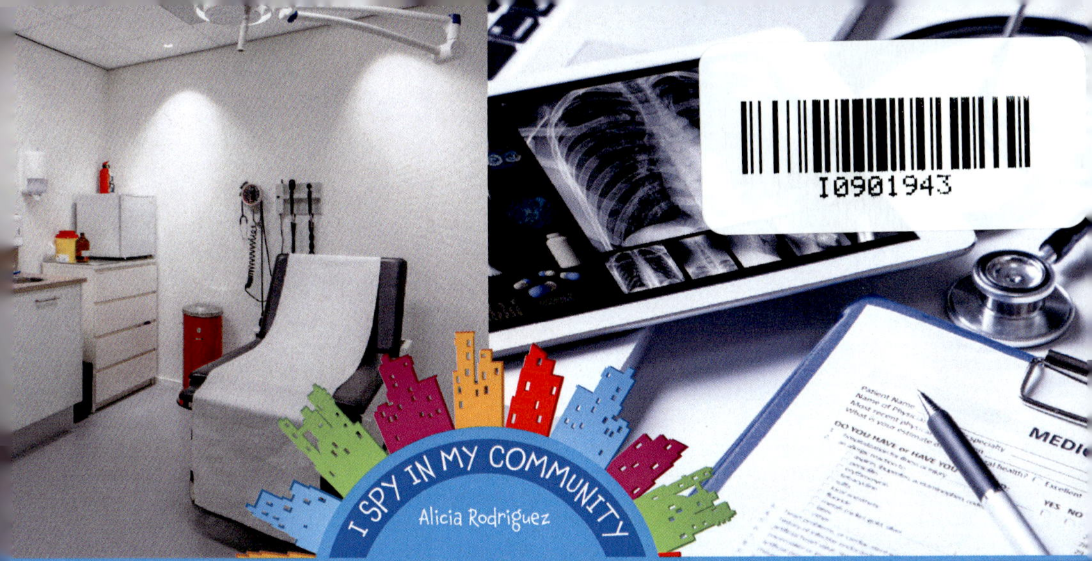

I SPY IN MY COMMUNITY

Alicia Rodriguez

DOCTOR'S OFFICE

A Crabtree Roots Book

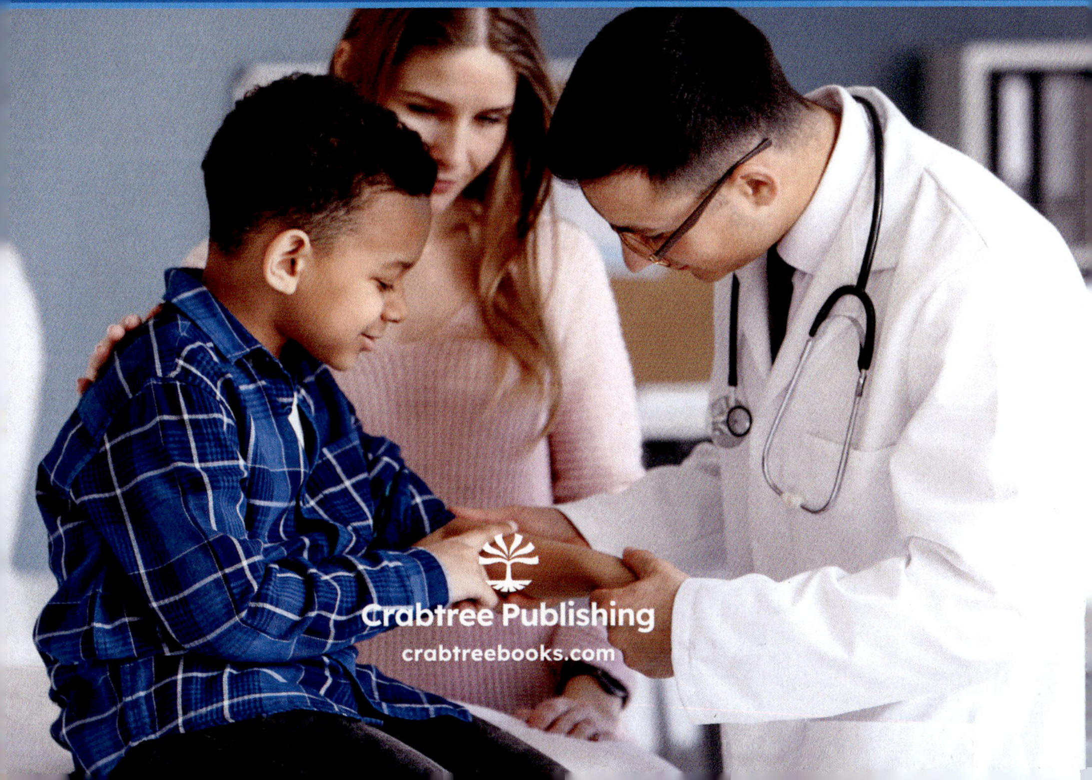

Crabtree Publishing
crabtreebooks.com

School-to-Home Support for Caregivers and Teachers

This book helps children grow by letting them practice reading. Here are a few guiding questions to help the reader with building his or her comprehension skills. Possible answers appear here in red.

Before Reading:

- What do I think this book is about?
    - *I think this book is about what a doctor's office looks like.*
    - *I think this book is about a doctor's office.*
- What do I want to learn about this topic?
    - *I want to learn what you can see in a doctor's office.*
    - *I want to learn how big a doctor's office is.*

During Reading:

- I wonder why...
    - *I wonder why the nurse checks my weight and height.*
    - *I wonder why the doctor listens to my heart.*
- What have I learned so far?
    - *I have learned that doctors can give people shots.*
    - *I have learned that the doctor can help me stay healthy.*

After Reading:

- What details did I learn about this topic?
    - *I have learned that doctors and nurses work at doctor's offices.*
    - *I have learned that doctors help people when they are sick or hurt.*
- Read the book again and look for the vocabulary words.
    - *I see the word* ***heart*** *on page 8 and the word* ***shot*** *on page 10. The other vocabulary words are found on page 14.*

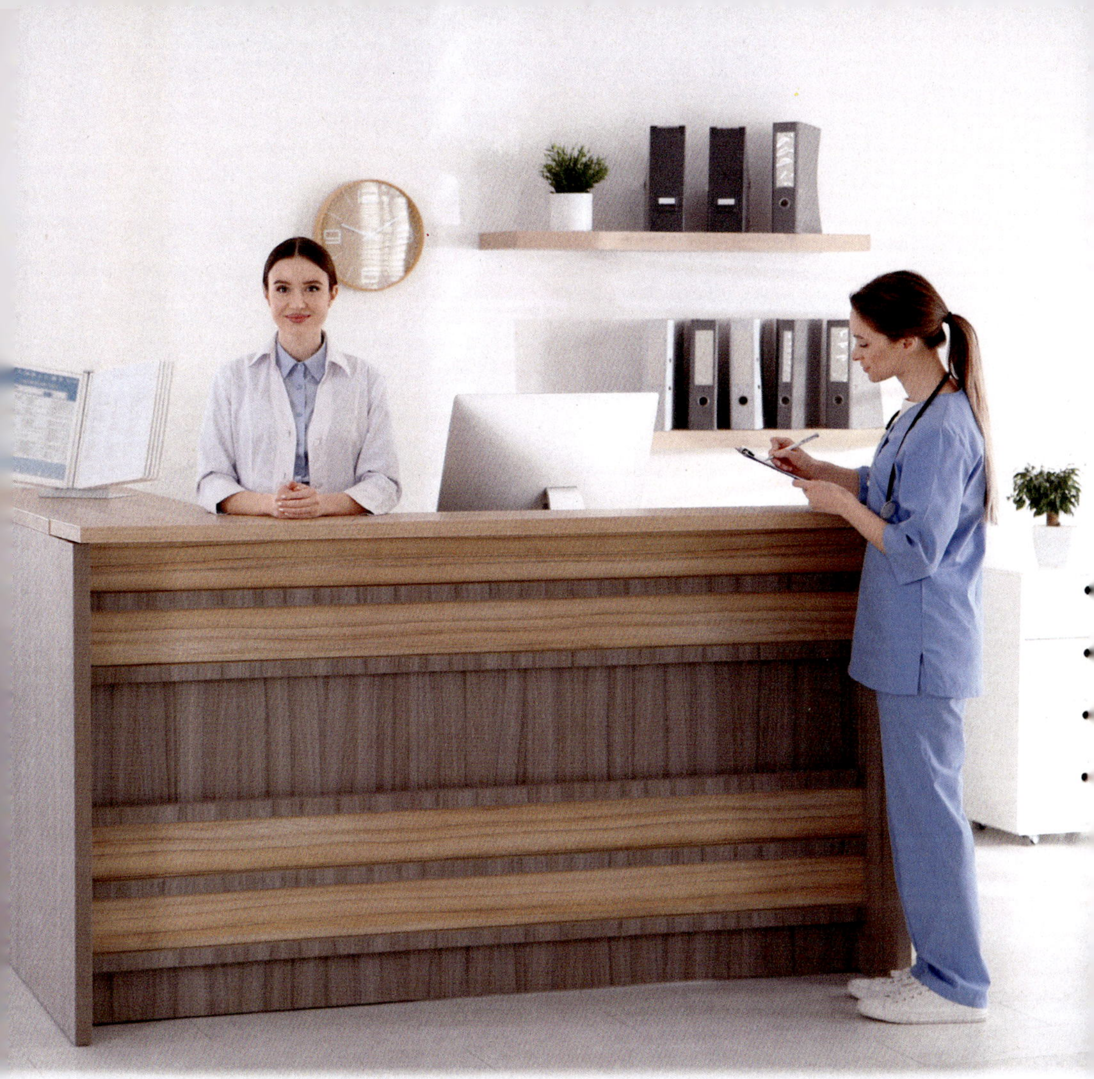

Time for my checkup at the **doctor's office**.

The **nurse** checks my weight.

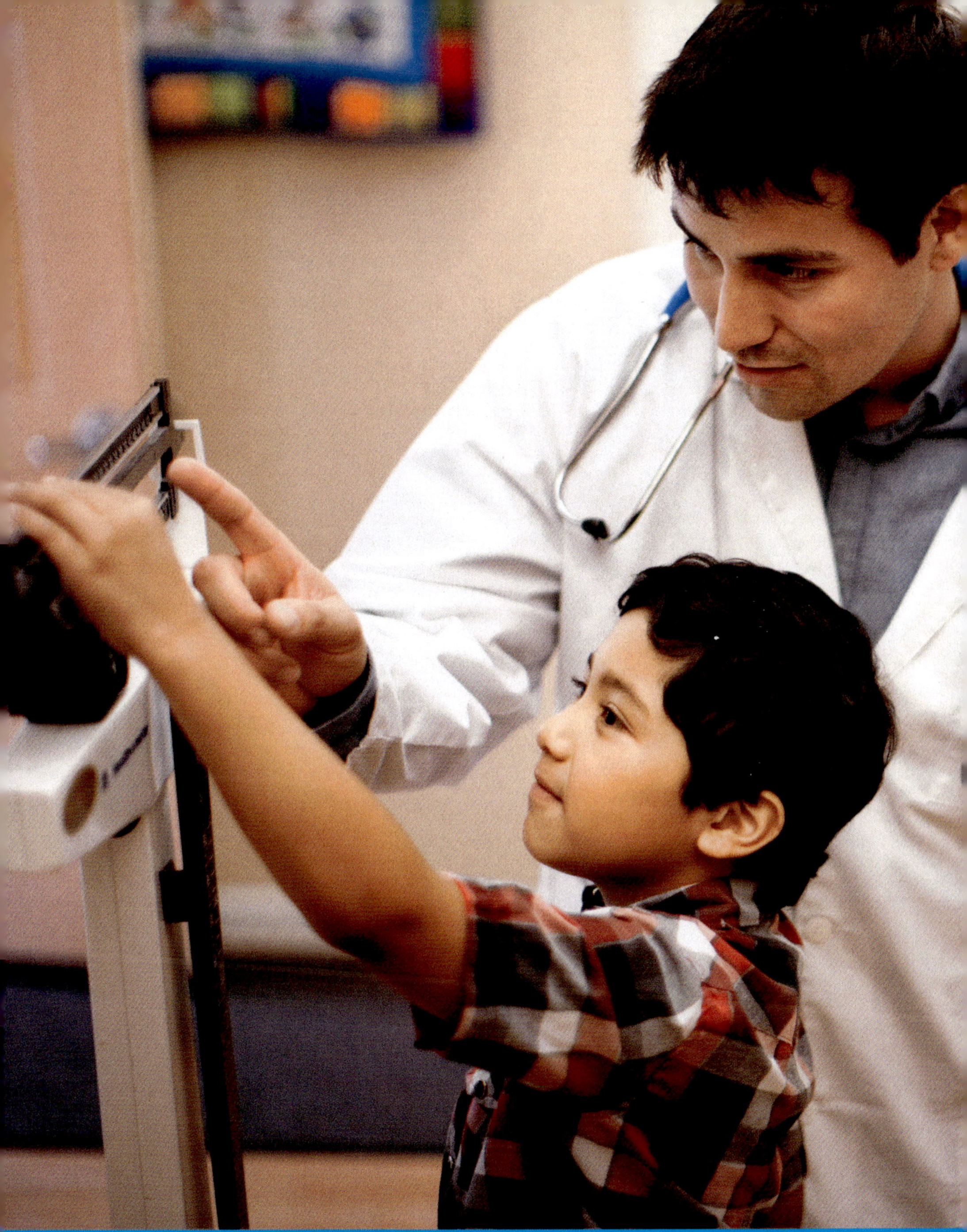

The nurse checks my height.

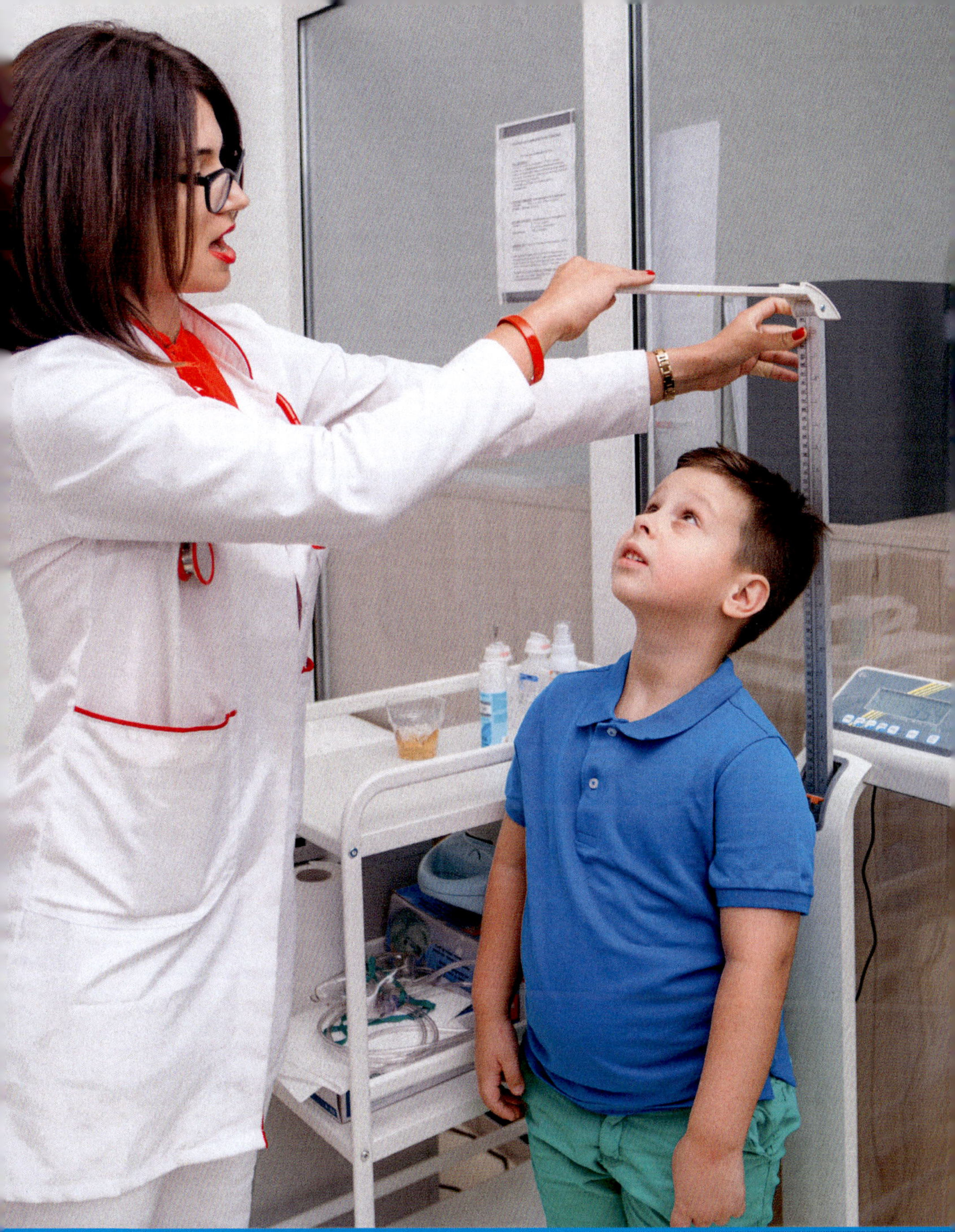

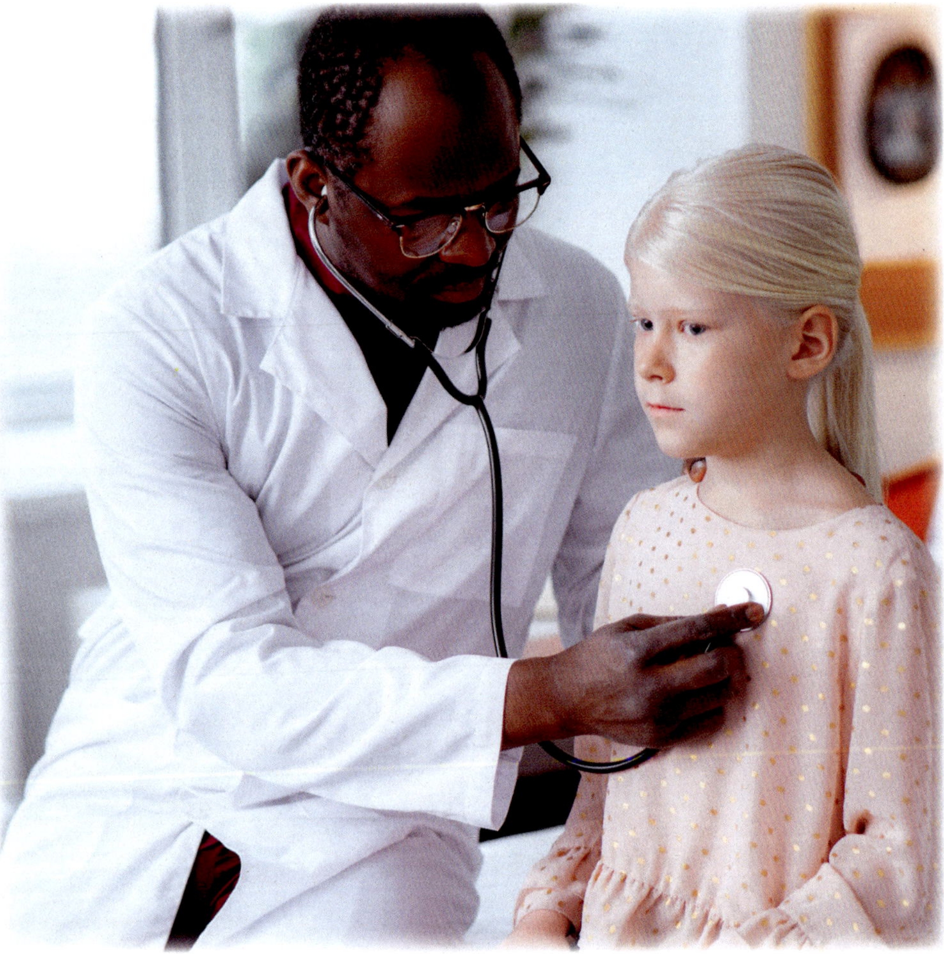

The doctor listens to my **heart**.

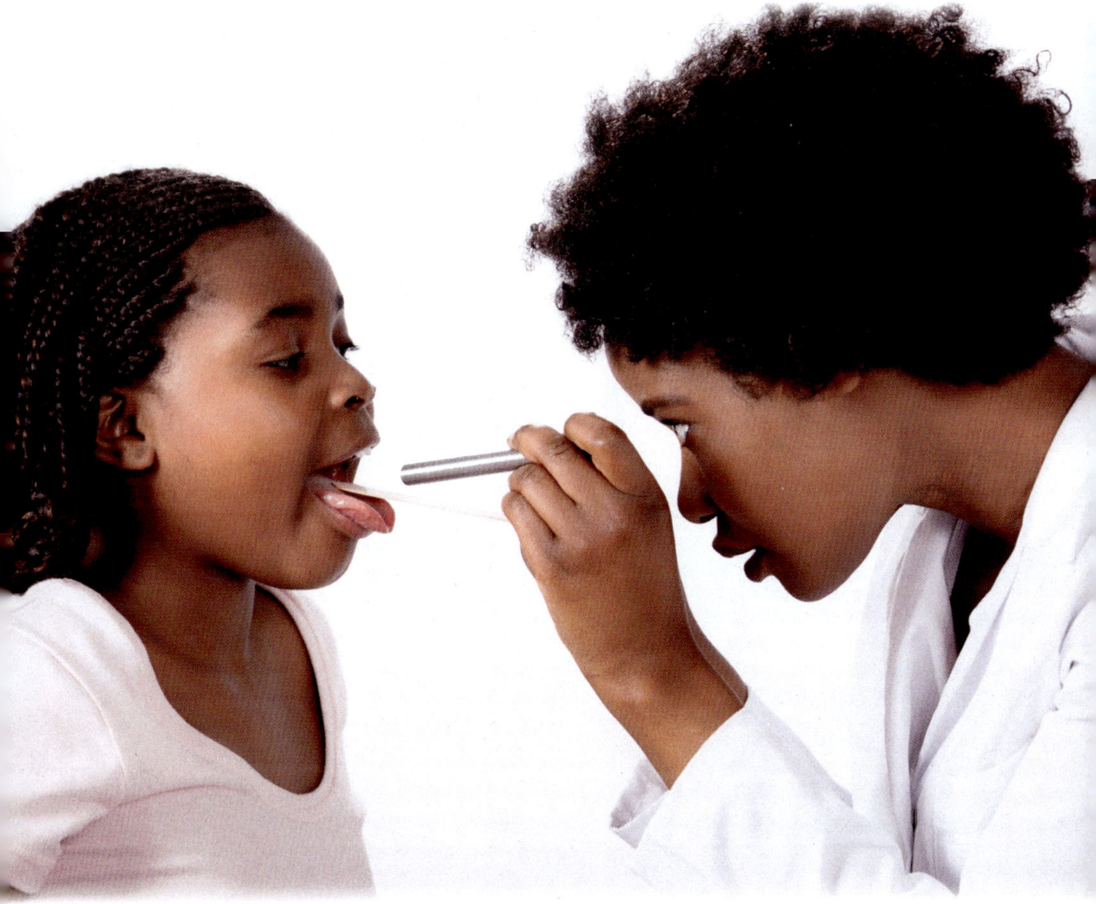

The doctor looks at my **throat**.

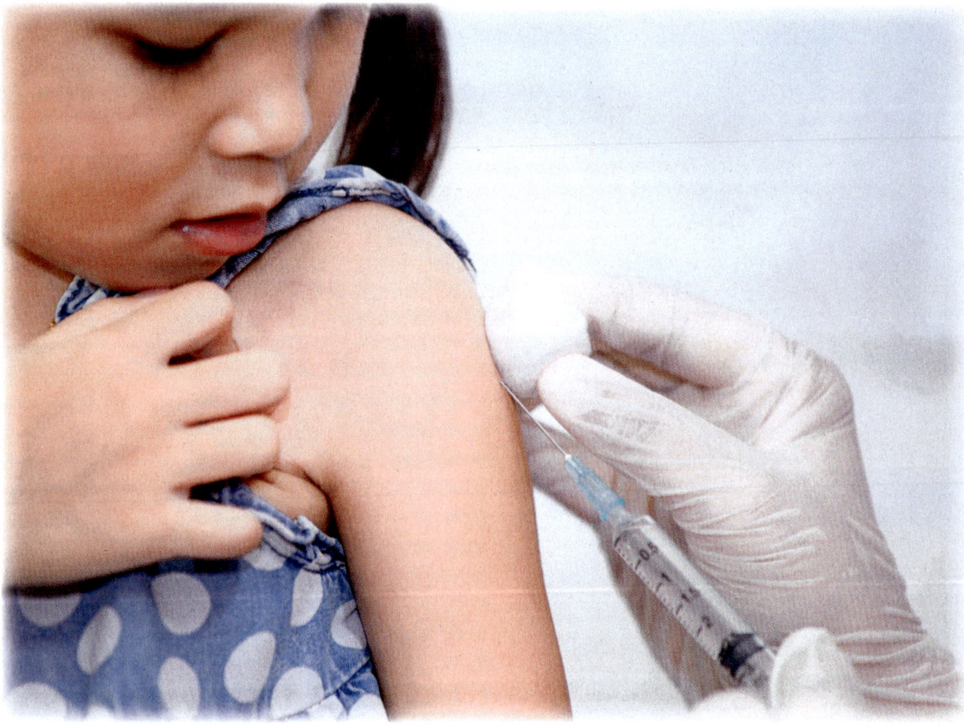

I am brave when I get my **shot**.

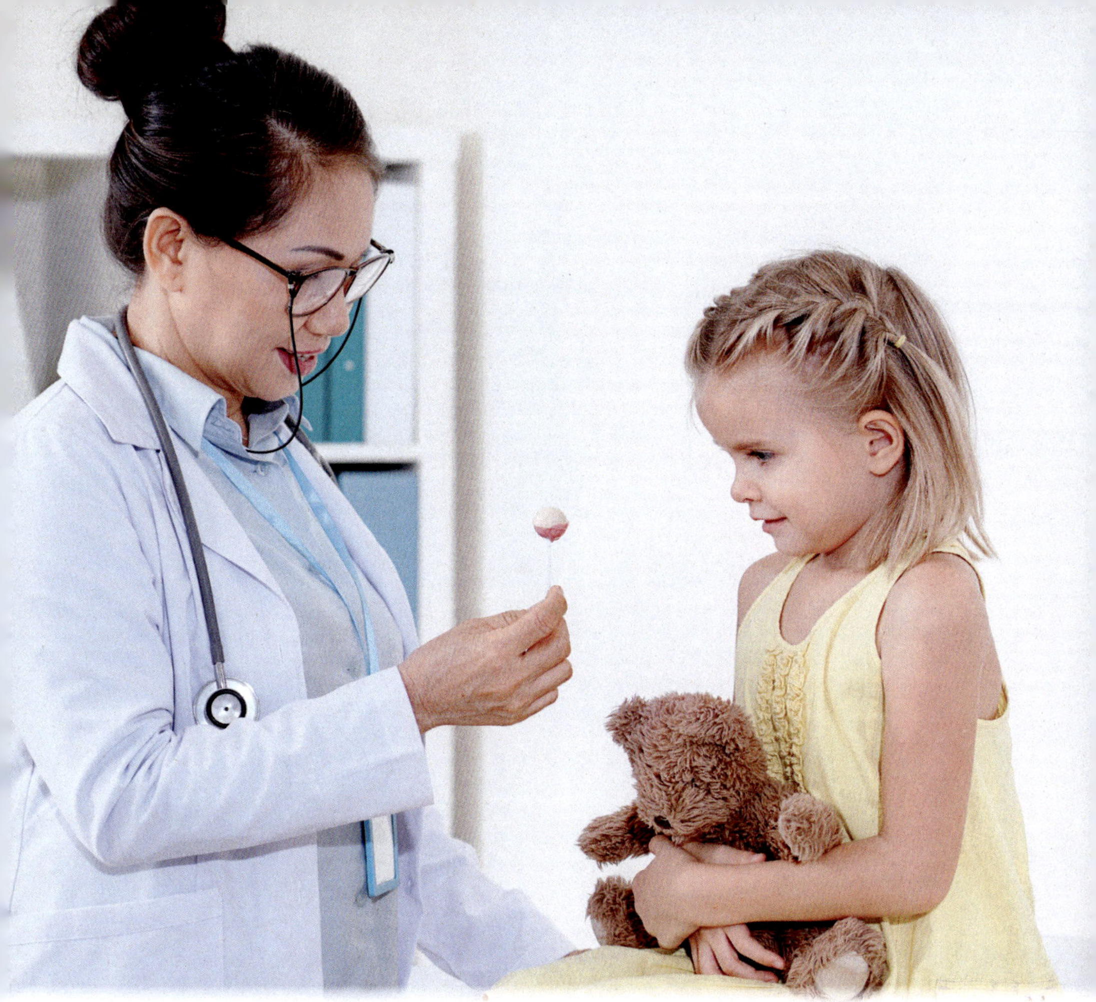

The doctor gives me a **lollipop**.

The doctor helps me stay healthy.

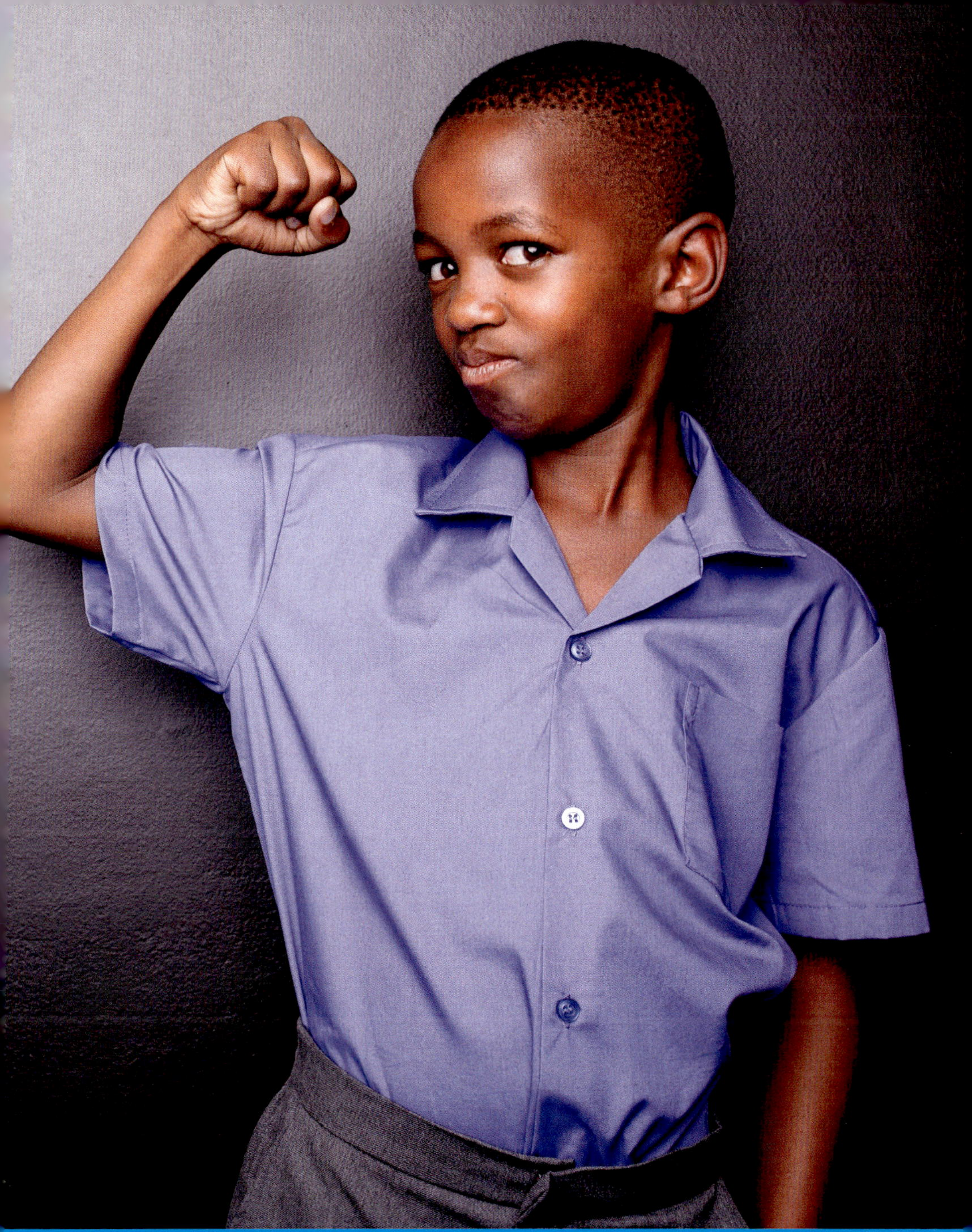

Word List

Sight Words

a
am
at
for
get
gives
helps
I
me
my
the
time
to
when

Words to Know

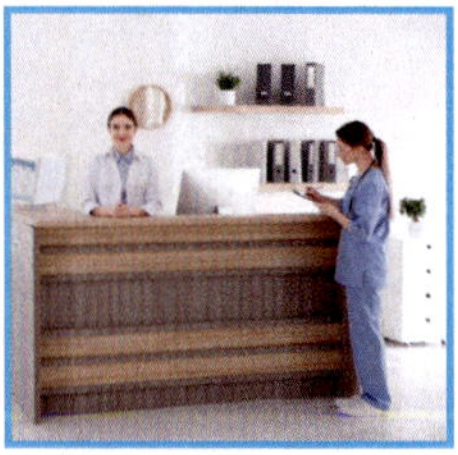

doctor's office

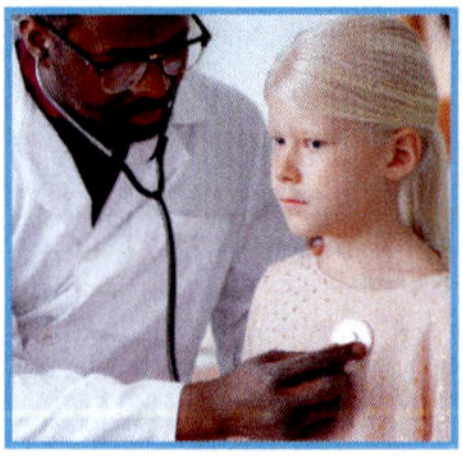

heart

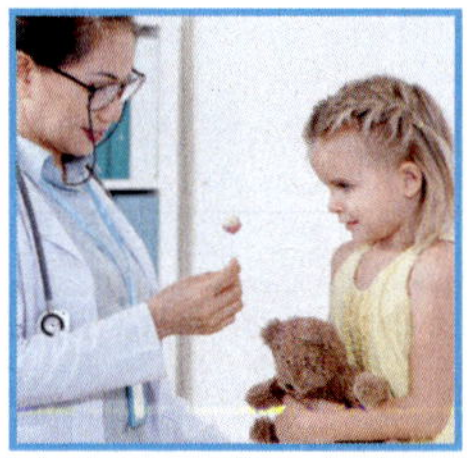

lollipop

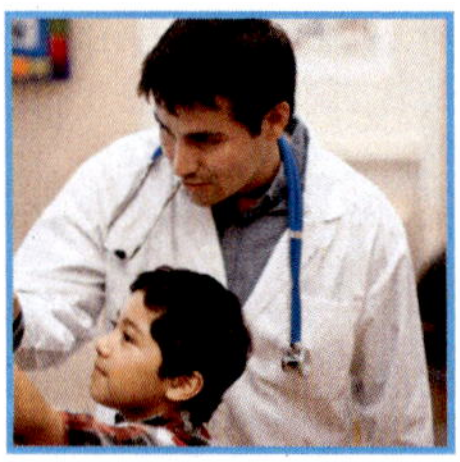

nurse

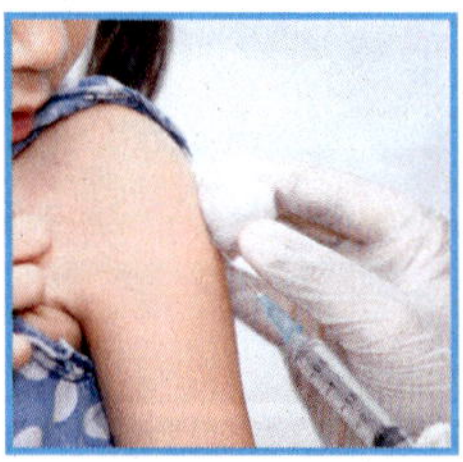

shot

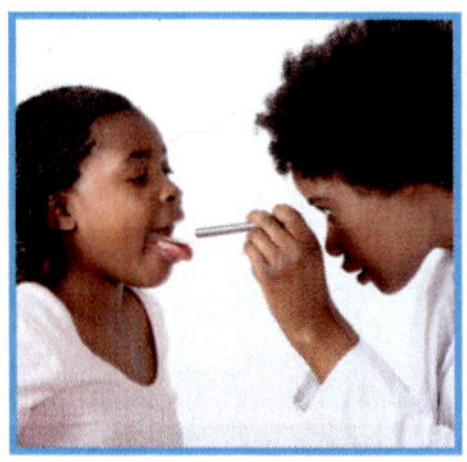

throat

50 Words

Time for my checkup at the **doctor's office**.

The **nurse** checks my weight.

The nurse checks my height.

The doctor listens to my **heart**.

The doctor looks at my **throat**.

I am brave when I get my **shot**.

The doctor gives me a **lollipop**.

The doctor helps me stay healthy.

DOCTOR'S OFFICE

I SPY IN MY COMMUNITY

Alicia Rodriguez

Crabtree Publishing

crabtreebooks.com 800-387-7650

In Canada: We acknowledge the financial support of the Government of Canada through the Canada Book Fund for our publishing activities.

Hardcover	978-1-4271-5723-2
Paperback	978-1-4271-5729-4
Ebook (pdf)	978-1-4271-3371-7
Epub	978-1-4271-3431-8
Read-along	978-1-4271-5747-8
Audio book	978-1-4271-5752-2

Library and Archives Canada Cataloguing in Publication
Title: Doctor's office / Alicia Rodriguez.
Names: Rodriguez, Alicia (Children's author), author.
Description: Series statement: I spy in my community | "A Crabtree roots book".
Identifiers: Canadiana (print) 20210197463 | Canadiana (ebook) 20210197471 | ISBN 9781427157232 (hardcover) | ISBN 9781427157294 (softcover) | ISBN 9781427133717 (HTML) | ISBN 9781427134318 (EPUB) | ISBN 9781427157478 (read-along ebook)
Subjects: LCSH: Children—Medical examinations—Juvenile literature. | LCSH: Medical offices—Juvenile literature.
Classification: LCC RJ50.5 .R63 2022 | DDC j610—dc23

Printed in Canada/042024/CPC20240422

Published in Canada
Crabtree Publishing
616 Welland Avenue
St. Catharines, Ontario
L2M 5V6

Published in the United States
Crabtree Publishing
347 Fifth Avenue
Suite 1402-145
New York, NY 10016

Written by: Alicia Rodriguez
Designed by: Rhea Wallace
Series Development: James Earley
Proofreader: Janine Deschenes
Educational Consultant: Marie Lemke M.Ed.
Photographs: Shutterstock: Byonkruud: cover (top left); Metamorworks: cover (top right); Pixelshot: cover (bottom); New Africa: p. 3, 14; Ericksonstock: 5, 14; Gorgev: p. 7; Yakobchuk Viacheslar; p. 8, 14; Andrey_popov; p. 9, 14; A3pfamily: p. 10, 14; Dragon Images: p. 11, 14; Nolte Image: p. 13

Library of Congress Cataloging-in-Publication Data
Names: Rodriguez, Alicia (Children's author) author.
Title: Doctor's office / Alicia Rodriguez.
Description: New York, NY : Crabtree Publishing Company, 2022. | Series: I spy in my community - a crabtree roots boo | Includes index.
Identifiers: LCCN 2021018042 (print) | LCCN 2021018043 (ebook) | ISBN 9781427157232 (hardcover) | ISBN 9781427157294 (paperback) | ISBN 9781427133717 (ebook) | ISBN 9781427134318 (epub) | ISBN 9781427157478
Subjects: LCSH: Medical care--Juvenile literature. | Medical offices--Juvenile literature. | Physicians--Juvenile literature.
Classification: LCC R130.5 .R64 2022 (print) | LCC R130.5 (ebook) | DDC 610--dc23
LC record available at https://lccn.loc.gov/2021018042
LC ebook record available at https://lccn.loc.gov/2021018043